THE HCG GUT CLEANSING

YOUR BASIS FOR DOUBLE SUCCESS IN YOUR METABOLISM CURE. WHY A METABOLISM CURE AFTER GUT CLEANSING IS MUCH MORE SUCCESSFUL.

FRANK SCHMIDT

ISBN 978-1-63920-153-2

Contents

Preface

Dear readers,

Tens of thousands of people have managed to reduce their weight with a metabolism cure, reaching a lower Set-Point[1] of their body thanks to HCG. That way they laid the foundation for sustainable weight reduction. I myself have lost over thirty kilos in the last year, and I gained some insights that as far as I know haven't been written down so far. But they increase the effectiveness of a metabolism cure and provide an even more sustainable success.

Through using the HCG intestinal cleansing, that is an intestinal cleansing program incorporating HCG, it is possible to on one hand increase the weight reduction induced by the metabolism cure. On the other hand the body is enabled to pick up vital substances much better.

I am publishing this progress report in order to inspire other people through my experiences. In this little booklet I will introduce you to an enhancement for the metabolism cure that by now many people will be familiar with.

Good luck with your weight reduction

Frank Schmidt

[1]Set Point is the weight that the body registers as "normal". It always strives to reach that weight.

ONE

THE MEANING OF INTESTINAL HEALTH FOR BODY AND MIND

The bowel brain, scientifically dubbed "enteric nervous system", runs through the entire abdomen. It contains about a hundred million nerve cells, which is about five times that of your spinal column. This independent nervous system comprises a thin layer between the muscles of the digestive system. The bowl brain controls the digestion and works autonomously. It does however interact with the entire organism. Or to say it in other words: What happens in our intestines has a much bigger impact on our whole body and our well-being than we would think.

It is not surprising then, that more and more providers of intestinal cleansing methods and products are crowding the market. They have understood one basic truth: An intestine covered in slag and putrefactive bacteria and containing faecal stones (faeces stored for a long time) cannot work well.

The reception of nutrients and vital substances is disturbed long-term, and sooner or later the body will poison itself. This will become apparent through various illnesses and ailments. Latest research has shown that there is a connection between periodontosis and intestinal health.[1]

The best strategy for sustainable health is very easy: As long as you don't have to fight acute ailments or illnesses, you should get to the root of it, which undoubtedly is in the intestines.

During my weight reduction I noticed quite early that a dietary program wasn't the proper way. I did lose weight with it, but that weight loss came with side effects that were unexplainable to me.

On some days I was losing weight quite well despite not really keeping to the diet plan, and on other days I didn't lose any weight despite keeping to it.

Additionally I was on the verge of becoming a "vacuum cleaner" for vital substances. It seemed to me that I could almost feel my money churning in my mouth in the form of pills and capsules. Since all in all I was still losing weight, I thought it was worth it. However, after I had gotten through the first phase of the diet, and decided to give my body some reast, I began getting a bit deeper into the topic. I noticed that the person who was supporting me in my dietary efforts had not properly, or not at all, explained important health aspects as well as the role of the intestine.

I am using compounds made by the company Lifeplus, which was recommended to me by a friend who had lost over thirty kilos with it himself, and all in all the products as well as the company itself looked very trustworthy to me.

That was a decision that I never regretted. However, I did regret that my friend who advised me on the topic didn't know a particular lot about it himself - other than when I should take which compound.

That is not really anything against the products, and not against the distribution concept of the company either. Even so, I think it is very important that people who give others advice and recommendations about health should actually have learned about the topic themselves, and should not just repeat what others said.

So, after I had lost my first 12 kilos within three weeks, I was regarding the topic "weight loss" in a new light. I wanted to know how it all worked. I found the entertainingly written book by Julia Enders[2]. In it she describes the "unknown creature" intestine that rumbles around in the abdomen and - as it seemed - does nothing but stink and create pungent waste products. Julia Enders had opened my eyes with her book, and I realised that I had to get to the root of all the evil. The intestines excrete substances (even the valuable vital substances that I was ingesting during my metabolism cure), and others.

In this book, I decided, I will describe the products and amounts I consumed, as well as my criteria and experiences. All that is a subjective report, and not an instruction to do the same thing. Furthermore I am neither a therapist nor a nutritionist. I am writing this booklet as a layman.

All bodies react differently. So what was good for my body might not be the right way for another's.

[1]Read: Peter Carl Simons: Chlorophyll - Gesundheit ist grün, 2015, BOD.

[2]Enders, Julia: **Gut: the inside story of our body's most under-rated organ, 2015**

TWO

GUT CLEANSING AS A DIETARY PROGRAM

My first access to the topic of intestinal cleansing was quite easy. I imagined what it would be like to fertilise my lawn with the best fertiliser in the world - but in winter, when the grass lies dormant under twenty centimetres of snow. Just a small portion of the fertiliser would even reach the ground, and the largest part would be swept away by melt water.

Our intestine works the same way when it's covered in slag, old faecal stones in intestinal pockets, putrefaction bacteria and fungi. Even the best nutrients full of vitamins and trace elements will turn into putrid mud in this environment that will rather hurt your body than help it.

So if I - staying with my lawn metaphor - have some patience, I would progress a bit smarter: I would uncover the grass, or wait until the snow has melted. Afterwards I just need a small fraction of that best fertiliser and it will still yield better results than fertilising grass under twenty centimetres of snow.

That was my strategy before tackling my next metabolism cure. I wanted to make my intestine as receptive as can be. How I did that, I will describe in the following text. Of course, in the context of intestinal cleansing, there are many important topics to be discussed. For one, there is the question about losing the slag substances and the faecal stones. Additionally I wanted to get rid of the parasites in my intestine. On this topic, Wikipedia.de reads:

Intestinal parasites mean the infestation of the intestine by parasites like worms (worm diseases) or protozoa (certain flagellates and amoebas). These parasites usually reach the intestine by smear infection, in which they may sometimes survive for quite some time. They cause unspecific ailments up to heavy diarrhoea (caused by entamoeba histolytica for example).

You might think I am heartless, but: I wanted to get rid of these little creatures, and I did.

Afterwards I tried to decrease the remaining toxic substances, and build up a healthy and balanced intestinal flora that will allow me to lose more than "just" a dozen kilos in the second metabolism cure. Naturally I wasn't primarily concerned with taking pills, but I wanted to focus on adjusting my diet – in a way that allowed the intestine to absorb vital substances ideally.

As this change in diet was, in my case, accompanied by a calory reduction, I used HCG again, based on my previous experience with the HCG metabolism cure. I will elaborate on that later.

THREE

THE USED ACTIVE SUBSTANCES

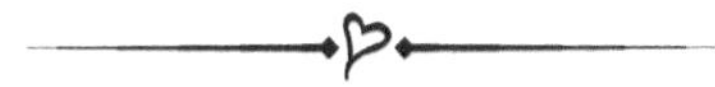

The following display of the vital and support substances I used is merely an experience report of what worked for me. The same thing is true for the named products.

Gut cleansing

The focus of every intestinal cleansing is the physical intestinal cleansing. I have divided that, for myself, in two concepts: I used Aloe Vera as a "cleaning agent", and a large supply of fibres to allow the intestine to optimise itself sustainably.

Aloe Vera is a beautiful plant, and its medicinal capabilities have been used for over 6000 years. Even the medicinal script *Papyrus Ebers* from ancient Egypt portrays Aloe Vera– also dubbed "plant of immortality" - as a remedy for bladder and intestinal issues.

The approximately 160 active substances in the plant are being deciphered very slowly. What made me decide for it was its active substance Acemanane. The substance is currently also being researched in the context of supporting cancer therapies. On the topic of intestinal cleansing, Peter Carl Simons states in his book[1]:

An intestinal cleansing effect is also documented, as well as a build-up of a healthy intestinal flora. That allows nutrients to be broken down and absorbed into the intestinal wall more effectively.

Through the increase in cell activity, Acemanane strengthens the immune system and makes the body defend itself more actively against parasites, viruses, bacteria and funghi. That is why aloe should always be part of intestinal cleansing methods.

For the intestinal cleansing I consumed two Aloe Vera caps from Lifeplus each, in the morning and in the evening. That is a bit more than the recommended daily dose, but it worked very well for me. The Aloe Vera concentrate in the caps is made from whole Aloe Vera leaves through a patented method. I think that is very important because most of the important ingredients of aloe, as in most plants, is "right under the skin". During the production of Aloe Vera gels, these ingredients are usually omitted.

Along with Acemanane, which by the way humans produce on their own until their puberty, the plant contains many vitamins, enzymes, amino acids and minerals that support intestinal cleansing.

The second part of my intestinal cleansing strategy consisted of the consumption of fibres. Their importance for intestinal health has been known for a long time. On the topic of fibres, Wikipedia.de states the following:

The fibres contained in chyme can bind water, and thereby increase its volume – chyme rich in fibres thus exerts more pressure on the intestinal wall and thereby supports preistalsis, shortening the dwelling time of foods rich in fibres (as opposed to the stomach) in the intestine.

No complex animal has enzymes for breaking up water-unsoluble fibreslike cellulose – the fact that these substances are still broken up for ruminants is largely attributed to the microorganisms living inside their rumen. In the small and large intestines, however, such bacteria do not exist, so that water-unsoluble fibres pass the digestive system practically unchanged.

(...)

Along with water, fibres also bind minerals, toxins, bile acids, as well as microorganisms that are subsequently excreted with the faeces. With a balanced and mixed diet that doesn't pose a problem, but additional fibre consumption can lead to a lack of mineral substances in the long term.

It was my plan to help my intestine, with intestinal cleansing (and renovation), to find its way back to its full functionality. I am convinced that our body is made to largely regulate itself, and to take all necessary actions. Due to a wrong diet, negative influences, and the increasing denaturalisation of our foods, however, it needed a little jump start.

For this jump start, however, I did not listen to the recommendation of my friend to use a Daily-Plus product of Lifeplus, but instead I used Colon Formula, from the same company. Simply put, it was the same product, with one difference – Daily Plus contained additional vital substances.

Vital substances are a good thing, of course. But as I had read in various articles, my body would simply excrete many of the vital substances that it cannot absorb in just a few hours, so I believed it made more sense to consume fibres – which I did only once a day – and vital substances separately, with the latter ones being consumed over the course of the day.

Every breakfast included a shake with two cups of the Colon Formula from Lifeplus. To give it some taste, I added some fruit juice to the water (100 percent natural).

Summary:

2 x 2 capsules Lifeplus Aloe-Vera-Caps (morning and evening)

1 x 2 cups Lifeplus Colon Formula at breakfast

Getting rid of parasites and toxins

It is well known nowadays that the human intestine, due to consuming a lot of bread and similar foods, tends to attract funghi. Heavily meat-eating individuals in turn attract putrifactive bacteria in their intestine. These are only two examples for what an imbalanced diet can do to our digestive tract. Additionally, for people who eat lots of unwashed fruit and vegetables, there is a higher risk for getting intestinal parasites.

When the intestine is out of balance, the putrid, partly inflamed, and parasite-laden intestine environment can produce toxins that are distributed throughout the body, leading to various diseases.

All the more important it became to me, to not only cleanse my intestines, but also to make sure that parasites are killed and toxins are excreted. On the Lifeplus website I found a product description for Lifeplus Paracleanse on the topic:

*The product Paracleanse is a synergistic combination of herbs and herbal essences, sulfuric amino acids, and MSM, thoroughly harmonised for the support of the interior cleansing of the body_*[2].

It was especially interesting that the product contained MSM, an important sulfuric compound for excreting toxins. In addition to the dose of MSM contained in Paracleanse, I consumed Lifeplus-MSM.

The thinking behind that idea was that I was already reducing my calory intake during my intestinal cleansing phase. The additional dose of MSM should help excrete the additional slag substances during the weight reduction. You can find further information on MSM in my book on the topic of HCG metabolism cure, as MSM is an important supporting substance for the metabolism cure.

Summary:

3 x 1-4 Pellets Lifeplus Paracleanse each day

3 x 1-5 Pellets Lifeplus MSM each day

(The chapter about the process contains a more in-depth description.)

Good basic supply – the beginning of everything

It is by now largely known that a proper supply with vital substances[3] is incredibly important for your health. Many of the fruits and vegetables we consume nowadays, however, contain far less vitamins, trace elements, etc., than they did twenty years ago. That means that a normal consumer can hardly keep up with the vital substance supply using normal methods anymore.

In order to make sure that the body absorbs the vital substances ideally throughout the day, I consumed TVM-Plus - two pills each, three times daily. By now they are part of my basic supply, as well as Lifeplus Proanthenols 100. Once you have used these two wonderful products and noticed their positive influence on your own well-being, you won't want to part with them anymore. I am convinced of that.

Summary:

3 x 2 Pellets Lifeplus TVM Plus each day

3 x 1 Pellets Lifeplus Proanthenols 100

Acid-base-balance

In her book "Der Basen-Doktor"[4], Maria Lohmann states:

When consuming too many acidic foods and carbohydrates, they cause fermentation processes in the intestines, as well as acidification and gas excess. A basic diet will support the intestine and the regeneration of the mucous layer. Smelling faeces and uncontrollable gas usually imply protein decay, while for fermentation processes the smell tends to be sour.

Naturally it was also my aim to, during the intestinal cleansing, regenerate my intestinal mucous layer. So I decided to also work on my acid-base-balance. The testing strip from Lifeplus showed me how my values developed.[5] In order to improve those values, Lifeplus PH Plus was ideal for me. An important part of its recipe is magnesium, and I had struggled with a lack of magnesium for years. This was often expressed through cramps in my legs, and trouble falling asleep. This product hit two birds with one stone.

Summary:

2 x 3 Pellets Lifeplus PH Plus each day

I began with 2 x 3, and briefly increased the dosage to 3 x 3, but went back to 2 x 3 pellets after reaching better test values. But as I already mentioned, every body reacts differently.

HCG – Reducing weight and keeping the new weight

The use of HCG for adjusting weight originates from the British physician Doctor Simeons in the mid-20th century. In India he observed pregnant women working in the fields, consuming little nutrients. Despite the lack of vitamins and the hard field work, they gave birth to healthy and well-developed children.

This was an amazing fact that Doctor Simeons researched in the following years, before he discovered the endogenous messenger substance HCG as well as its effect inside the human body. HCG positively affects the hypothalamus, which is part of the interbrain. The hypothalamus controls hunger and the feeling of satiety.

This control centre acts in accordance with our own set-point. The set-point theory states that every human has his very own "normal value" for his weight. The body tries to keep this exact weight. That explains why some people can keep their weight under any circumstances, but it also shows why some people experience a re-increase in weight after a successful diet (the so-called yo-yo-effect).

The hypothalamus can be compared with a thermostat. It perpetually checks whether the current weight is the same as the set-point. If it is not, the body undertakes measures to adjust the weight. Through consuming HCG, the set-point itself can be altered, as long as the treatment takes at least 21 days.

As the intestinal renovation requires an adjusted diet anyway, and less calories are taken in during that diet, I decided to secure my success by simultaneously using homoeopathic HCG drops. The activation of my metabolism was a positive side effect of the HCG. My body now burned more calories and dissolved fat stores "in the right places". Additionally, the compound decreased the feeling of hunger.

Summary:

3 x daily, one unit of HCG

Various manufacturers offer these as drops, globules or as a salt – the recommended dosages usually work quite well.

Diet adjustment

Other than with the HCG metabolism cure, which focuses on weight loss, my focus for the HCG intestinal cleansing was treating my intestine to all the best things I could. I did that with two simple methods:

Carbohydrate-reduction

Carbohydrates, and bread and similar products especially, lead to growth of funghi in the intestines. That is understandable, as making bread from grain is a relative novelty in human history. The roughly ten-thousand years in which humanity has systematically baked bread weren't enough for their bodies to adjust completely. That makes it logical that our intestine doesn't exactly have a method for handling these relatively unknown substances. Due to that reason, I completely omitted baked goods from my diet during the whole intestinal cleansing process (and even today I try to consume as little of it as I can). As I additionally aimed at more weight loss, I also tried to avoid carbohydrates where I could. Reputable nutritionists nowadays agree that the body doesn't break down fat as long as it has carbohydrates to burn. That means fats are stored. And that's what I wanted to avoid.

Fat reduction

Fats increase the putrifactive bacteria in the intestines, but I wanted to get rid of those. This quote by Peter Carl Simons shows how important this is for optimising the whole body:

Nowaday's research shows that gingival pockets secrete sulcular fluid. It is a waste product from the intestines that travels through the blood. Reputable scientists assume a correlation with putrifactive processes in the intestine, and have found that inflammations – especially with the support of chlorophyll – are reduced in many cases with intestinal renovation.[6]

Common sense tells us that it makes little sense to fight the consequences of malnutrition with great effort, when those efforts at the same time "feed" the perpetrator. That is why I deliberately ate little fatty foods during my intestinal cleansing phase. This means the amount of fat in the foods as well as the low-fat preparation of them. A "nice piece of meat" loses a lot of fat when it's prepared on a grill or a contact grill instead of a frying pan. Additionally this helped with my secondary goal, the weight loss.

As the use of HCG kept my feeling of hunger low, I designed my diet in the same way as for a metabolism cure. Instead of a dieting phase I incorporated thirty days of intestinal cleansing into my metabolism cure. The two harmonised perfectly. During that month I lost another twelve kilos, while obtaining a "freshly cleansed intestine".

It is also important to leave at least four hours between the main meals and other food consumptions.

[1]Peter Carl Simons: Aloe Vera – 6'000 Jahre Medizingeschichte können sich nicht irren, 2015, BOD

[2]http://lifeplus.com/us-de/product-details/6117)

[3]Wikipedia.de: "Vital substances are vital ingredients working as bio catalyzers in cells and tissues with water, oxygen and carbon dioxide (in plants). They include: Enzymes, co-enzymes, hormones, exogenically essential amino acids, exogenically essential fatty acids, main and trace elements, scent and taste substances."

[4]Lohmann, M.: Der Basen-Doktor, 2013, 2nd issue, Trias

[5]If the testing strips show an acidic value, that means that our body is excreting excess acid, which is good. But if we lower our acid balance altogether, the body has to excrete less acid, which is even better.

[6]Peter Carl Simons: Chlorophyll – Gesundheit ist grün, 2015, BOD

FOUR
THE PROCESS

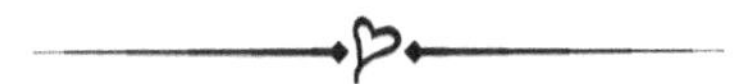

My intestinal cleansing was planned around one month. There are suppliers who offer programs for two weeks or less, but I personally don't trust those. Things that have been going wrong over the course of several years can't be fixed in a healthy way in two weeks in my opinion. This is why I wanted to give my body enough time, especially to excrete parasites and toxins.

Blow you will find a table of the products I used. It shows the products that were successful for me. This does not represent a treatment advice, and in no way a "health promise".

Lifeplus Aloe-Vera-Caps

2 x 2 Capsules (in the morning and the evening each)

Lifeplus Colon Formula

1st week	1 tea spoon dissolved in water or juice, before the meal
2nd week	2 tea spoons...
Starting with the 3rd week	3 tea spoons

Lifeplus Paracleanse

3 x 1-4 Pellets a day (1st - 16th day)

1st day	3 x 1 pellets
2nd day	3 x 2 pellets
3rd day	3 x 3 pellets
4th - 16th day	3 x 4 pellets
Afterwards	omit

Lifeplus MSM Plus

3 x 1-5 Pellets a day

1st - 3rd day	3 x 1 pellets
4th - 6th day	3 x 2 pellets
7th - 12th day	3 x 3 pellets
12th - 16th day	3 x 4 pellets
17th - 30th day	3 x 5 pellets

Lifeplus TVM Plus

3 x 2 Pellets a day (Morning / Noon / Evening)

Lifeplus Proanthenols 100

4 x 1 Pellets a day (Morning / Noon / Evening)

Lifeplus PH Plus

2 x 3 Pellets a day (Morning / Noon / Evening)

HCG

3 x Daily, 1 portion according to manufacturer information

FIVE

OPTION: INTESTINAL CLEANSING WITHOUT LOSING WEIGHT

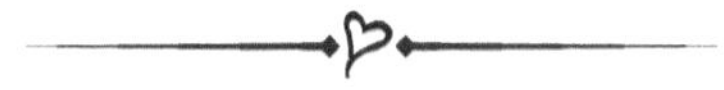

My colleague Anton asked me if he could conduct intestinal cleansing without losing weight. Other than me, he doesn't have a weight problem. We had a long discussion about how he could proceed best. In the end, he was successful with the following method:

Anton went through the steps "intestinal cleansing", "getting rid of parasites and toxins", "basic supply" and "acid-base balance" the same way I did. However, he did not take HCG. And during the diet adjustment he avoided bread and bread products (processed grain), but otherwise consumed sufficient carbohydrates (rice, potatoes, pulses, fruit). This way he managed to limit his fat consumption.

During his intestinal cleansing, Anton only lost one kilo, which afterwards he gained back rather quickly. That way he could keep his desired weight.

Based on Anton's experience I believe the approach is viable for people without weight problems as well. Underweight should not become an issue. But as I already mentioned: I am no nutritionist or medical practitioner. Please consult an expert on dietary adjustments.

SIX

WHAT IS THE NEXT STEP

As previously mentioned, I started my stabilising phase of the HCG metabolism cure directly after my HCG intestinal cleansing. This was possible because I was already following the menu plan of the diet phase of an HCG metabolism cure during the intestinal cleansing.

For me personally, I decided to conduct an intestinal cleansing at least once – or better twice – a year. Whether I will include HCG or not will depend on whether or not I want to also reduce my weight (I currently don't have my "dream measurements").

The consumption of the basic vital substances Lifeplus Proanthenols and Lifeplus TVM Plus, as well as Lifeplus Omegold[1] 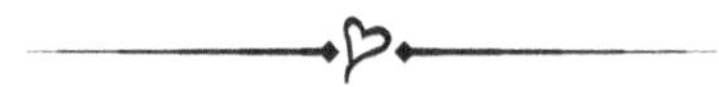 was aimed at achieving an ideal basic supply. I also want to generally keep my reduced consumption of baked goods and carbohydrates. I do, however, think that it makes more sense to "kick over the traces" once in a while.

All in all I buy groceries in a more planned and deliberate way. When in doubt I prefer to buy lean meat, and to prepare it with little fat.

[1]This substance was not shown in this book. You will find annotations about it in my work about the HCG metabolism cure.

SEVEN

CONCLUDING NOTES

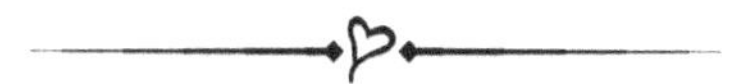

All statements made in this book are to be seen as an experience report. They are no medical consultation, nor are they a recommendation for imitation. In general, I have merely reported my own experiences. I cannot speak for other people or make any promises on the effects or on a cure.

The products and companies mentioned in this text are within the context of an impartial report. The statements were not discussed with the manufacturers or other representatives. I also deliberately avoided using the names of the products and companies in an advertising way, but I simply used their common name on the market.
My statements are not a scientific evaluation. I do not explicitly claim that the products used are better or worse than products made by other manufacturers.

The described vital substances can be acquired from any Lifeplus-Partner. If you do not know a source, or if you want to post feedback on this book, please contact me directly at:

Please note that I am no nutritionist, medical practitioner or healer. That means that I cannot consult you personally via email or telephone, but if you wish, I can recommend people to you who can.

Bibliography

- Auer, Dr. med. W.: Übersäuerung – die stille Gefahr, 2002, Kneipp-Verlag
- Arndt, U.: Spirulina, Chlorella, AFA-Algen: Lichtvolle Power-Nahrung für Körper und Geist, 2003, H. Nietsch
- Bachmann, Dr. med. R. M.: Natürlich gesund durch Säure-Basen-Gleichgewicht. Mit Ihrem persönlichen 7-Tage-Programm zur sanften Entsäuerung, 2001, Trias, 2. Auflage
- Bankhofer, Prof. H.: Aloe Vera: Die Pflanze für Gesundheit, Vitalität und Wohlbefinden, 2013, Kneipp-Verlag, 6. Auflage
- Barcroft, A.: Aloe Vera: Nature's Silent Healer, 2003, Baam
- Beringer, Alice: Aloe Vera – Die Königin der Heilpflanzen: Natürlich gesund und schön durch den reinen Extrakt der Aloe Vera, 2007, Heyne
- Berner, H.-G.: An vollen Töpfen verhungern, 1997, Medi Verlagsgesellschaft
- Bertram, Dr. K.: Spirulina – Die Wunderalge – Anbau, Vorkommen und Zucht, sensationelle Studienergebnisse, Krankheiten vorbeugen und bekämpfen, o. J., CreateSpace
- Bisel, Ch.: Ich war ein fetter Sack: Wie ich einfach, schnell und ohne Hungergefühl über 30 Kilo abnahm – und wie Sie das womöglich auch können, Bisel Consulting, 2014
- Bisel, Ch.: Das BMI-Coach Ernährungstagebuch: Das Erfolgs-Tagebuch für Ihre Diät zum Wunschgewicht, Bisel Consulting, 2015

- Bisel, Ch.: Die BMI-Coach Stoffwechselkur: Ihr Weg zur nachhaltigen Gewichtsreduktion bis hin zu Ihrem Wunschgewicht, Bisel Consulting, 2015
- Dahlke, R.: Fasten Sie sich gesund – Das ganzheitliche Fastenprogramm, 2004, Irisana
- Dahlke, R., Ehrenberger, D.: Wege der Reinigung – Entgiften, entschlacken, loslassen, 2002, Heyne, 2. Auflage
- Delbé, J. B.: Gesund werden – gesund bleiben: Aloe-Vera-Leitfaden Gesund bleiben, 2004, M+M Verlag
- Enders, J.: Darm mit Charme, 2014, Ullstein
- Finnegan, John &, Schmid, Rainer: Aloe Vera – das Geschenk der Natur an uns alle, 2014, Ernährung & Gesundheit, 35. Auflage
- Frauwallner, A.: Was tun, wenn der Darm streikt? – Probiotika sinnvoll einsetzen, 2012, Kneipp-Verlag
- Gill, T.: Lieber schlank als sauer – Gesund ins Gleichgewicht mit der Säure-Basen-Diät, 2012, CreateSpace
- Gray, R.: Das Darmheilungsbuch – Gesundheit durch Kolon-Sanierung, 2011, Trias
- Grillparzer, M.: Simple Detox: Das 7-Tage-Entgiftungsprogramm, 2013, Gräfe und Unzer, 5. Auflage
- Jester, F.: Arginin. Der natürliche Kraftstoff für Blut, Kreislauf und Gesundheit, 2010, Verlag Marina Jester
- Jester, F.: Chlorophyll. Das grüne Blut, Verlag Marina Jester, 2014
- Kraske, Dr. med. E.-M.: Säure-Basen-Balance, 2008, Gräfe und Unzer, 5. Auflage
- Liebke, Dr. F.: Doktor Chlorella! Die Alge fürs Leben. Kompendium zur Mikroalge Chlorella, Remerc & Lheiw verlagskontor, 2007
- Loede, P.: Schlank mit Weizengras: Die Gruene-

Smoothie-Weizengras-Kur, CreateSpace, 2014
- Lohmann, M.: Der Basen-Doktor. Basische Ernährung: gezielte Hilfe bei den häufigsten Beschwerden, 2013, Trias, 2. vollst. überarb. Auflage
- Meyer, Marianne E.: Sonnenkraft mit dem blaugrünen Lichtträger Spirulina, 2002, Windpferd, 2. Auflage
- Mutter, Dr. J.: Grün essen!: Die Gesundheitsrevolution auf Ihrem Teller, 2013, VAK, 3. Auflage
- Opitz, Ch.: Befreite Ernährung, 2013, H. Nietsch, 5. Auflage
- Oppermann, J.: Aloe Vera – Was die Pflanze wirklich kann, 2004, Lebensbaum
- Peuser, M.: Kapillaren bestimmen unser Schicksal: Aloe – Kaiserin der Heilpflanzen, Quelle für Vitalität und Gesundheit, 2010, St. Hubertus
- Rahn-Huber, U.: Spirulina & Chlorella: Gesund und fit mit Mikroalgen, 2015, Riwei
- Rahn-Huber, Ulla: Natürlich heilen und pflegen mit Aloe Vera, 2015, Riwei
- Schneider, G. W.: Biotop Mensch – Liebe Deine Darmbakterien, 2014, Biotop Mensch, 7. Auflage
- Simons, C. P.: Aloe Vera - 6'000 Jahre Medizingeschichte können sich nicht irren, 2015, BOD
- Simons, C. P.: Chlorophyll – Gesundheit ist grün, 2015, BOD
- Simons, C. P.: Grüner Kaffee – Garantie zum Abnehmen, 2015, BOD
- Simonson, B.: Gerstengrassaft: Verjüngungselixier und naturgesunder Power-Drink. Wildpferd, 15. Auflage, 2012
- Simonson, B.: Die Heilkraft der Afa-Alge – Vitalität für Körper und Geist, 2000, Goldmann
- Skinner, R.: Aloe Vera: The Medicine Plant, 2005, Mill Enterprises

- Skousen, M. B.: Aloe Vera Handbook: The Acient Egyptian Medicine Plant, 2005, Book Publishing Company
- Thust, Th. M., Schlett, Dr. med. S.: Entgiften & entschlacken,
- 2006, Gräfe und Unzer
- Treutwein, N.: Übersäuerung – krank ohne Grund?, 2005, Weltbild
- Ulmer, G. A.: Gesundheitswunder Chlorophyll: Gespeicherte, gesundheitsspendende Sonnen- und Heilkraft, Ulmer, 1997
- Vollmer, J. B.: Gesunder Darm, gesundes Leben, 2010, Knaur
- Wacker, S., Wacker, Dr. med. A.: 300 Fragen zur Säure-Basen-Balance, 2013, Gräfe und Unzer, 2. Auflage
- Wagner, W.: The Chlorophyll Supplement: Alternative Medicine for a Healthy Body, 2013, Health Collection
- Wolfe, D.: Superfoods – die Medizin der Zukunft: Wie wir die machtvollsten Heiler unter den Nahrungsmitteln optimal nutzen, Goldmann, 2015

www.ingramcontent.com/pod-product-compliance
Lightning Source LLC
Chambersburg PA
CBHW021148260726
48656CB00025B/2271